Sleep on It!

Sleep on It!
Waking up to the Importance of Sleep

Essays and Practical Commentaries
from the
Pedagogical Section Council of North America

Published by
Waldorf Publications at the
Research Institute for Waldorf Education

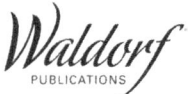

Printed by:
Waldorf Publications at the
Research Institute for Waldorf Education
351 Fairview Avenue Suite 625
Hudson, NY 12534

Copyright ©2025
by the Pedagogical Section Council of North America

Title: *Sleep on It! Waking up to the Importance of Sleep*
Editors: Liz Beaven and Holly Koteen-Soulé
Front cover: *Infusion*, painting by Ursula Stone, with permission
Back cover image: Anouk Tompot
Layout: Ann Erwin
Proofreader: Luke Stence
ISBN# 978-1-963686-09-8

Contents

Introduction 1
  Elizabeth Beaven

Ten Questions about Sleep 3
  Betty Staley

Sleep and Rhythms 8
  Florian Osswald

Drawbridge and Porticullis: Thresholds of
Sleeping and Waking Consciousness 14
  Douglas Gerwin

Rest as Resistance: A Social Aspect of Sleep 24
  Linda Williams

Healing Forces of the Night 28
  Holly Koteen-Soulé

Sleeping to Awaken: Sleep and Social Change 36
  Vernon Dewey

Sleep and the Chronology of Transformation 43
  Vernon Dewey

Sleep and Movement 48
  Laura Radefeld

Resources for Further Exploration into the Nature
and Significance of Sleep...................... 50
   Michael Holdrege

Mission and Membership of the Pedagogical Section
Council of North America..................... 52

Introduction

Elizabeth Beaven

This booklet is the result of several months of research and discussion by members of the Pedagogical Section Council of North America. Members took up a study of the important and somewhat mysterious role of sleep in human life and in education. Each member explored a different aspect of our study and that work formed the basis for the following chapters. We are fortunate to also include observations by Florian Osswald, former co-director of the Pedagogical Section at the Goetheanum, on this topic.

In his preparatory work with the teachers of the first school (Stuttgart, 1919), Rudolf Steiner stated that a fundamental task of the teacher is to teach the children to sleep and breathe in a healthy way. On first encountering this statement, many of us have pondered its significance and meaning. It is a theme and task that Steiner returned to again and again in this first course and in other lectures on education and human life. It is also a theme that has gained increased notice within Waldorf education and, more broadly, in society and medicine, as we see the serious effects of insufficient sleep and sleep disruption reported almost universally by teachers today. Steiner was well ahead of his time in emphasizing the significance of healthy sleep; he remains ahead of our time in his emphasis on the role of education and the educator in developing it.

What, exactly, did Steiner mean? How do we impact our students' sleeping and awakening? Why does this matter? What are the roles of sleep and dreams? What do the many references to sleep in mythology tell us? What do we give students during the day to enrich their sleep lives? How do we prepare for and "harvest" the fruits of the night? How can movement support healthy sleep? What about our own sleep? What practical strategies could we implement for ourselves and our students? How can we support our work with the healing and strengthening power of sleep? These questions, and more, are addressed in the following pages from the perspectives of anthroposophy and contemporary research. Some of these essays explore the nature of sleep and waking primarily from social or spiritual perspectives. We trust that you will find them helpful as we all continue to study and better understand what Steiner meant in giving us this primary task.

This booklet is dedicated to Betty Staley (1938–2025), a member of the Pedagogical Section Council for 40 years, student of Rudolf Steiner and Waldorf education for 57 years. Fittingly, she developed a series of questions on sleep for our consideration.

Ten Questions about Sleep

Betty Staley

Experiencing healthy sleep is a challenge for most people today, including parents, children, adolescents, and also teachers. Since we spend about one-third of our lifetime in sleep, it is important to strive for the best quality of sleep and get it at the right times. It is as important to our survival as food and water. Recent research shows that a chronic lack of sleep increases the risk of serious disorders including high blood pressure, cardiovascular disease, diabetes, and obesity, as well as depression.

Teachers need energy and clear thinking, along with stamina, to meet the needs of the children. Every day teachers are called upon to prepare their lessons, carefully observe children, and be alert to what the children are needing. From a scientific point of view, if we can't form or maintain the pathways in our brain that let us learn and create new memories, then it is harder to concentrate and respond quickly. These pathways are built and strengthened during sleep. If teachers arrive at school already exhausted, how can they be at their best?

The following questions are directed to our fellow teachers to help us be more conscious of how to achieve healthier sleep.

1. How do you prepare for sleep? What is your routine? Do you have a practice that helps you prepare? Do you avoid caffeine and nicotine late in the day and alcoholic drinks before bed? Is the computer or TV located in your bedroom or is it in a separate place? What are your thoughts as you prepare to put away the day's activities and turn to the night? Have you been off the screen for at least an hour or two before you turn in? Do you wind down before bed with a warm bath, reading, or some other relaxing routine?

2. Do you have trouble falling asleep? Once you are in bed, do you toss and turn, remembering things you forgot to do, wondering whether you have prepared properly for tomorrow's lesson, or asking yourself whether you answered a child's need during the day, or concerned about a conversation you had with a parent? How can you enter sleep ready for rest?

3. What images are you carrying into sleep? For example, if you are concerned about a particular student, what image do you have of that student? Picture scenes during the day going back to the morning when you had your first interaction with the student. Do you have an image of the student's facial expression, of what clothing they were wearing, of how they interacted with classmates? How does that make you feel? Are you interested in knowing more about the student? Can you open your heart so that you feel a flood of love surrounding the student? Can you carry that love into your sleep?

4. What questions do you carry into sleep? Are there questions you put to the spiritual world? For example, how can I prepare my class so that it inspires the children to have stronger imaginations of the characters presented in class? Or, what do I need to do to stimulate Johnny's interest in the lesson? Perhaps your questions have to do with your colleagues: How can I be more open and sympathetic to one or more of my colleagues? Why does a particular colleague always frustrate me?

5. What happens when you decide to "sleep on" a problem? It has become common knowledge among sleep experts that the importance of getting a good night's sleep cannot be overstated when you are having a problem in life or at work. They suggest that you analyze the problem and its possible solutions, then sleep on it before making a final decision. Some suggest you sleep on it for three nights before making the decision. For example, the neuroscientist Matthew Walker, in his book *Why We Sleep*, describes how different kinds of sleep help us solve problems. The dreaming state that most typically occurs in REM (rapid eye movement) sleep helps us process emotions, develop insight, and work socially with others, while the NREM (non-rapid eye movement) sleep works more with memory and information and promotes creativity.

6. How do you work with the memory of colleagues or others who have passed away? Rudolf Steiner gave many lectures about life after death. If we are open to the possibility of being able to communicate with souls who have crossed the threshold of death, our relations with departed souls can also be a source of help to us in our lives and work. Through posing questions to departed colleagues or family members before going to sleep, we may find impulses coming to us at the moment we awaken or at different times of the day.

7. How can you work with a colleague or parent as you prepare for sleep when you have had misunderstandings? It is helpful in this case if you can spend a few minutes focused on this person before sleep. Can you feel interest in the person, create an image of the person, and ask what that person's life is like? What is that person's goal in this situation? How would you behave if you were that person? Offer up an image of the person to the night and see what comes in the morning.

8. How is your sleep readying you for the next day? What is your pattern of awakening? Do you wake up to the sound of an alarm clock and spring out of bed? Do you wake up slowly, taking time to listen to what comes to you from sleep? Try to be quiet and listen. If you have a notebook nearby, you can jot down some thoughts before you join the bustling of the day.

9. What do you give your children to carry into sleep? Although the earlier questions have to do with the teacher's sleep, here we turn to the sleep of the children or students. The stories, the activities, and the work the children do during the day all carry over into sleep. What messages have they taken from these activities? Is there a message of how human beings can care for one another? Are there examples of bravery, of sacrifice, of true dignity? During the next day in class, pay attention to the children's comments about the previous day's lessons. What images do they carry from the previous day that are revealed as you lead a review?

10. How can you work with sleep when you are teaching adolescents? Teachers need to understand that adolescents have a different circadian rhythm from their younger siblings. They get tired later in the night, long after their parents have gone to bed, and they need more sleep in the morning. Requiring teenagers to wake up at 7 a.m. and function well in their classes is a problem for most high schoolers. Adolescents try to deal with this discrepancy by using caffeine to stay awake. If you are giving the students an exam, they should have a good night's sleep rather than stay up late cramming for the test. It is more effective to divide the contents of a course into parts and test the students along the way than to give them a final exam that is asking them to remember back to the beginning of the class.

These ten questions can serve as a stimulus to research and discussion as teachers come to understand the powerful importance of sleep in our lives. These and other questions will be taken up in further detail by other members of the Pedagogical Section Council in their various contributions exploring Rudolf Steiner's indications on sleep.

And if tonight my soul may find her peace
in sleep, and sink in good oblivion,
and in the morning wake like a new-opened flower
then I have been dipped again in God, and new-created.

– D.H. Lawrence, "Shadows"

Sleep and Rhythms

Florian Osswald

Three polar activities determine people's lives in a special way: breathing in–breathing out, waking up–falling asleep, and being born–dying. Every age, every culture, and every individual assigns a meaning to these moments in life. In everyday life, they appear as silent companions. If we become aware of them, our relationship to them changes. For example, shortness of breath, sleep disturbances, or the anticipation of a birth or death can quickly become the focus of our attention and trigger strong feelings.

The relationship among these three "pairs" is not immediately obvious. A closer look, however, reveals a similar structure. The processes of being born, waking up, and breathing in represent a complementary change of consciousness to the moments of dying, falling asleep, and breathing out. We breathe in for the first time when we are born and breathe out for the last time when we die. In poetry, falling asleep is sometimes depicted as a small death and waking up as a small birth. With inhaling-exhaling or waking-falling asleep, the rhythmic structure is obvious, whereas in being born–dying it is only an assumption.

In *The First Teachers' Course*, given in 1919, Rudolf Steiner emphasizes the importance of these rhythms for education:

We must educate and teach, and bring harmony to the relationship between the children's breathing and the spiritual world. Human beings are unable to achieve the rhythmic change between waking and sleeping in the spiritual world as they can in the physical world. Our teaching and educating must bring harmony to this rhythm so that the living physical body can become well integrated into the spirit-soul.[1]

Breathing and sleeping as tasks of education? How can this be understood and, above all, implemented in the classroom?

Self-awareness can help with this. Breathing exercises already have a long tradition. Less well known are exercises connected with falling asleep and waking up. Sleep in particular still remains a riddle. Steiner gave a clue to this. In a lecture on October 10, 1918,[2] he describes an exercise for reviewing the night with a kind of retrospective that entails the following steps:

• Shortly after waking up in the morning, pause for a moment for a brief review of the morning so far, of the night, and of the previous evening. Imagine yourself going backward in time to the moment when you woke up. Perhaps you can see yourself getting dressed, brushing your teeth, pushing the duvet back, or opening a window.

• Go back one more step. Now you meet a kind of threshold. Keep going backward "into the night" as it were. Perhaps you remember a dream. Usually we do not have any memory of our sleep, it happens subconsciously.

• Keep going backward until you arrive at the moment you fell asleep. What were your last thoughts, your last feelings before falling asleep?

- Keep going backward for a few more moments into the evening and then stop.

This exercise focuses attention on the period of sleep, which still remains a riddle. Notice that the exercise does not start directly with the sleep phase, but with the transitions between falling asleep and waking up. As these steps take form, they can gradually help us get to know the mysterious in-between area better.

Interestingly, parents accompany their children into sleep as a matter of course, whereas we don't seem to pay much attention to ourselves when falling asleep. The exercise restores this attention by looking back on the day's events or asking a question of the "night." After waking up, looking back on sleep helps us to observe the effects of sleep. Teachers may describe, for example, how a song briefly introduced into a lesson can be easily recalled the next day or how a physics experiment can be almost completely forgotten on the following day.

Many questions arise here. Falling asleep has a lot to do with letting go and forgetting the experiences of the day. What can be happily forgotten and what not? As teachers, we can ask ourselves how we should organize the content of our lesson so that it is easily forgotten during the day in order to be processed well during sleep. Studying our own learning, forgetting, and remembering—incorporating our time asleep in this process—gives us an initial experience of this. We can also extend the sequence of night-time gaps and observe how something we have learned lives within us for two, three, or more weeks. Whatever happens, the memory content reveals something about the way in which it was taken up and worked on. The spectrum of memory will range from "precise" to "completely forgotten."

This self-awareness brings us closer to the main lesson or modular "block" form of teaching and clarifies our view of its effect. The question is how knowledge has developed during the gaps between the modules. Knowledge falls asleep and then we wake it up again. What significance does preparing for sleep have for waking up? What is helpful for a good awakening? The exercise starts with self-development but also opens up a new dimension of learning.

The third rhythm—of birth-death—is of course known to us but plays only a subliminal role in education. Newborns represent the archetype of a beginner. But they are not the only ones. At every age we have the opportunity to be beginners. In this sense, humans are the true beginners. And we also have the possibility to prepare ourselves for dying, because these two thresholds of our physical existence unconsciously determine our actions. Not knowing where I come from and where I am going creates a subliminal fear of life. In the words of Matthias Claudius, "If you don't die before you die, you die when you die."

How do we deal with these three rhythms? Indeed, what *is* a rhythm? It is not a beat, not a periodic recurrence of the same thing, not a repetition. Maldiney formulates it aptly when he says that moments of rhythm exist only in mutual relation to each other, in their unpredictable occurrence. Rhythm cannot be held "in front of you"; it does not belong to the order of owning or "having." We *are* in rhythm. Being present in it, we discover our presence within it. We live in this opening by living it. For Maldiney rhythm is a form of life, of existence as surprise.

Those who work with Steiner's pedagogical indications will pay attention to these three rhythms and cultivate and become increasingly aware of them in the course of the child's development. This is a great task and it opens new doors. We suddenly discover the three rhythms in many different areas of life. For example, children in many schools start the day by reciting the Morning Verse given by Steiner for the upper elementary grades. It begins with the line: "I look into the world..." and in the second part: "I look into the soul...."[3] The children look into the world and perceive it; they look into the soul and see what they think. This addresses a rhythm of perception and thinking that the children are made aware of every day. School life will connect them more and more with these two realms and articulate for them how they constitute their own activity. Individual aspects of the world are perceived with the senses and thinking brings them together to form a whole. Perception and thinking are a *fourth* rhythmic process.

In the context of the other three rhythms, perception is akin to falling asleep into the world. We arrive at a pure perception when the world speaks to us. In other words, we do not perceive what we already know, but what we do not know. Thinking in its purest form means awakening from out of the spiritual world, being newly reborn, bringing new knowledge into the world. In the Morning Verse, the children say: "The World-Creator weaves in sunlight and in soul-light." Here we live in pure vision. The world is a unity and reveals itself in two different forms: in perceptions and in the content of thinking.

If education is really to serve humanity and the world, then its foremost task must be to develop these four rhythms in age-appropriate ways.

ENDNOTES

1 Rudolf Steiner, *The First Teachers' Course*, GA 293/294/295, trans. Margot Saar (Bangkok: Plus Press, 2020), p.25.

2 _____, *Die Ergänzung heutiger Wissenschaften durch Anthroposophie*, GA 73 (Zürich, 10 October 1918). An online translation of this lecture is available here: https://rsarchive.org/Lectures/GA073/English/CMP2004/19181010p01.html Also Rudolf Steiner, *Anthroposophy Has Something to Add to Modern Sciences*, GA 73, trans. Anna Meuss (Clagiraba, Australia: Completion Press, 2004).

3 _____, Morning Verse for the upper classes, in *Toward the Deepening of Waldorf Education* (Hudson, NY: Waldorf Publications, 2017), p.117.

Drawbridge and Portcullis:
Thresholds of Sleeping and Waking Consciousness

Douglas Gerwin

In the course of a day we cross countless physical thresholds—stepping through an open archway from one room to another, opening or closing the door of a car or bus or train, entering or leaving a school classroom or office. In some cases, a door may open and close by itself; in other cases, you may need to push it open or shut it behind you, probably with no more than a fleeting glance of attention.

Falling asleep and waking up represent two further thresholds we cross at least once each day. But these transitions are markedly different in one key aspect. When you put your hand or shoulder to a door or simply stride through a doorjamb, you are likely to be focusing more on where you're headed than on where you've come from. By contrast, in the case of falling asleep and even waking up, the situation is the opposite: As we enter sleep, we have no preview of what to expect; likewise, as we approach the moment of awaking, we generally have no idea of what awaits us until we have actually crossed over into wakeful consciousness. Indeed, if we awaken in a strange bed or unfamiliar setting, for a moment we may lack even a sense of where we are. When it comes to sleeping and waking, we row backward, so to speak, across what the Ancient Greeks knew to be the dark River Lethe separating wakeful from sleeping existence.

Sometimes the threshold separating these two states of being may be experienced as blocked off, slowing or even preventing a smooth passage into or out of sleep. Already a century ago, Rudolf Steiner warned of an advancing epidemic of sleep disturbances, and recent surveys document an alarming rise in the number of people who struggle these days to fall—or stay—asleep or who may need an alarm clock or other sensory stimulant to return to wakefulness. Last year the U.S. Centers for Disease Control and Prevention reported that some 40% of adults surveyed stated they were not periodically but *chronically* sleep-deprived.

To recognize why a smooth transition from waking to sleeping may be disrupted, we need first to understand what is happening when we cross this threshold under normal circumstances. Here we come up against an initial problem: The very crossing of this threshold coincides in most cases with a total loss of daytime consciousness. Unlike stepping across a daytime threshold, in which we can typically anticipate what's ahead before we pass through it, at night we typically become aware of having crossed into sleep and then back into wakefulness only after the fact. How often have I inadvertently fallen asleep in bed while reading a book, discovering I had dozed off only after the book had slipped from my hand and crashed to the floor with a startling thud!

Put differently, the experience of falling asleep (and, perhaps to a lesser extent, also of awakening) is not subject to our control. As we rightly say, we "slip" or "fall" into sleep; we do not "step" or "leap" into it. Indeed, to capture the exact moment of passage into and return from a state of sleeping is simply beyond the reach of human awareness.[1] What is it, then, that draws us—or on occasion fails to summon us—across this threshold?

In one of his more provocative statements on this subject, Rudolf Steiner says we don't wish to sleep because we are tired but rather, to the contrary, that we grow tired because we wish to sleep—that is, we long to re-enter the spiritual world unencumbered by the constraints and exigencies of our living physical organism. In fact, he suggests our experiences during sleep are far richer than our waking experiences, since the latter are bound by the limitations of our physical body. Because we have not as yet developed the requisite organs needed to remember our spiritual journey during sleep, we generally cannot retain upon awakening any recollection of the experiences we had while asleep.[2] Even the dreams we have as we transit in or out of slumber easily vanish once we awaken.

Drawing upon his own spiritual research, Steiner offers some remarkably detailed descriptions of what happens to a healthy adult between the moments of falling asleep and awakening, whether from a quick nap or from an extended period of repose.[3] Based on his fourfold image of the human being, he describes that, while our physical and etheric bodies remain united during sleep, our astral body and "I" free themselves from their living physical vehicle and enter into lofty spiritual realms.[4] In more common language, we say that during sleep we are "out of it": In this phrase, the "it" refers to our living physical organism, and being "out" implies transcendence beyond the physical world.

Lest this description be taken too simplistically, Steiner offers a much more nuanced picture. As one anthroposophical nurse once described it for me, during waking hours, our "I" and astral body are concentrated *within* the upper portions of our living physical organism (primarily our nervous and fluid systems) but simultaneously *around* our lower portions (such as the systems of metabolism) like a lemniscate, with the upper loop closed off within the upper region of our physical organism and the lower loop sweeping about us in the lower region, a bit like a hoop skirt. In sleep this relationship is "involuted" or turned inside out and upside down: While "I" and astral body are released from within the upper portion of our living physical organism, in their higher forms they dive all the more deeply into our lower abdominal and autonomic muscular systems. It's as though our own "I" and astral body need to get out of the way "upstairs" so that our higher self as well as other higher cosmic beings can work their restorative genius on our sleeping organism from out of "downstairs." As our "I" and astral body lift out above in sleep, so "a divine astral body and ego are seen clairvoyantly to flow in [below]. The [human] body becomes the bearer or temple of higher Beings who guard and protect it. This divine astral body and ego are in fact active also by day, but are then overpowered by our own."[5]

To complete this picture: Between these two complementary opposite poles of our living body resides a middle realm of heart and lungs, which never tire since they never fully sleep nor fully wake. And yet even in these organs, especially in our lungs, we can experience a radical shift of activity as we slip into sleep. Notice how the breathing changes in sleepers once they "check out." As Rudolf Steiner describes it, when we are awake and inside our body, we draw air into our lungs by a process akin to suction; when we sleep, our "I" and astral body now push air into our lungs, as it were, from without by a process comparable to pressure, like bellows blowing air into a bonfire.[6] Breathing becomes deeper, often louder. Though we may occasionally sigh or snort during the day, only at night do some of us engage in steady snoring!

As suggested earlier, obstacles of a physiological, psychological, and spiritual nature may disturb, even block the transitions into and out of sleep. Some obstacles are well documented, especially those of physiological origin such as excesses of sugar (indeed drugs of any kind), light (both natural and artificial, as for example from digital screens), or rigorous muscular exercise shortly before bedtime. Other obstacles of a more psychological nature, such as emotional burdens or the excitement of anticipation (the night before a family celebration, for instance), will also be familiar.

Rudolf Steiner points to disruptions or imbalances of a more spiritual nature, however, that may go undetected. Adults prone to being too caught up in the world of the spirit may have difficulty taking hold of their bodily instrument and as a result are insufficiently awake during the day; they never quite make it "in" to their body, as it were. Consequently, they may lack sufficient hunger to return to the spiritual world at night since they never quite left it. Put differently, the best preparation for leaving one's physical organism at night is to have intensely occupied it in full wakefulness during the day. By the same token, those prone to being overly attached to the physical or material world may lose sight of their spiritual origins and in consequence may unconsciously tamp down the inbuilt yearning to return to it. For them the prospect of sleep can become tainted with a dimly felt sense of repugnance, impatience, even dread. Either way, the end result may be an obstructed entry into sleep.

However, if we are able to return in sleep to the spiritual worlds from which we emanate—as well as to welcome visitation by higher beings to the temple of our sleeping physical body while we rest—we accomplish three crucial tasks of healthful development while asleep: We grow, we heal, and we learn.[7]

From another point of view, one can compare the transitions of awaking and falling asleep to the periods of twilight between bright daytime consciousness and dark nighttime consciousness, or what D.H. Lawrence liked to call "our deepest lower…blood-consciousness."[8] On this view, the passage across the twilight threshold from waking to sleeping at dusk, for instance, can be greatly helped by feeling a calming mood of *trust* in the spiritual world, confident that it can imbue us with the healing and strengthening powers we need to remedy the consequences of the day past and to prepare us for the demands of the day to come.

The practice of Epimethean *gratitude*—for matters both cosmic and quotidian—helps lower the drawbridge to sleep; along with Steiner's oft-recommended *Rückschau* or bird's eye retrospective of the day just concluded, one can also try brief exercises of movement that include actually taking a few steps backward toward the bed so as to enhance this sense of trust in the as-yet unseen world of sleep. In fact, this happens naturally when we turn to sit down on the edge of a bed or couch.

As for the advent of dawning wakefulness, we need the warming mood of *courage* in order to pass safely beneath the daunting spiked portcullis that overhangs the transition from sleeping to waking. Here practicing upon awakening a brief exercise of Promethean *forethought* may be helpful before we actually open our eyelids, draw apart the curtains, and prepare to embrace the demands of the day. As Rudolf Steiner puts it:

> On days when something important is to happen to us we do not wake up exactly as we do on days that take their usual course—only we do not notice it. Those who used to lead the life of peasants on the land—such people knew about these things and did not like to be

torn suddenly out of sleep, because when there is no gradual transition into the waking life of day, one is wrested from such intimate experiences. Peasants say that on waking one should never look immediately at the window but away from it, so that while the light is still dim one can become aware of what is emerging from sleep... The more aware they become of that indefinite, half mystical influence which can radiate from sleep, the more clearly is their attention directed to their karma.[9]

In many cultural traditions, the transitional moments of twilight—dusk and dawn—are revered as a sacred or meditative time when the temporal and the earthly brush up against the eternal and the cosmic. As the sun falls asleep each evening beyond the curve of the western horizon, the vast planetary and starry realms of the spirit gradually come into view. But as the "rosy dawn," accompanied by Venus the Morning Star, heralds the return in the east of the radiant daytime sun, the star-studded celestial firmament dissolves into a period of invisibility. In this precious twice-daily transition, we are granted a fleeting glimpse of dynamic realms normally inaccessible to direct experience.

ENDNOTES

1. Florian Osswald, in a brief essay included in this collection, offers some simple yet challenging exercises to shed at least a glimmer of light on this transition into and out of sleep. In addition, there is a growing body of empirical research on what happens to our bodies as we fall asleep and as we prepare to wake up. See, for instance, *The New York Times* bestseller *Why We Sleep: Unlocking the Power of Sleep and Dreams* by Matthew Walker (New York: Scribner, 2017).

2. The reason for this amnesia, according to Steiner, is that in order to remember an experience, we rely upon the forces of our etheric organism, which however needs to remain with our physical body when we rest.

3. For a summary of Rudolf Steiner's many indications on this process, see his collection *Sleep and Dreams: A Bridge to the Spirit*, edited and annotated by Michael Lipson (SteinerBooks, 2003) or *The Wonders of Sleep: An Anthroposophical Study*, compiled and edited by Richard Seddon and Jean Brown (Wynstones Press, 2015). A comprehensive collection in German of Steiner's comments on sleep was prepared by Stefan Leber and published as *Der Schlaf und seine Bedeutung: Geisteswissenschaftliche Dimensionen des Un- und Überbewussten* (Verlag Freies Geistesleben, 1996). These indications describe an adult journey; the process is different for children up to the time of puberty.

4. Students of Rudolf Steiner's human anthropology will be familiar with his depiction of the fourfold human being:
   a) a physical or material body imbued with
   b) life forces (sometimes called etheric or vegetative body) and
   c) consciousness (named astral body or body of desire) as well as
   d) self-awareness ("I" or ego).

   A human being deprived of its "I" remains conscious but is not self-aware; a human further deprived of its astral body remains alive but no longer conscious; a human body deprived of its etheric forces is simply a lifeless material corpse.

5   Richard Seddon and Jean Brown, eds., *The Wonders of Sleep: An Anthroposophical Study* (Stourbridge, UK: Wynstones Press, 2015), p.59. As mentioned in the introduction to this collection of essays, we are all most grateful to my colleague Anouk Tompot, former Waldorf high school biology teacher, for creating and allowing us to use her drawing as the cover for this booklet. Though she had other ideas in mind when she fashioned this illustration, it serves to represent with elegant simplicity the relationship described here of "I" and "astral body" to the etheric body and physical organism in both waking (red) and sleeping (blue) conditions.

6   As with any such description, we use spatial terms (appropriate to picturing the physical material world of three dimensions) to characterize a non-spatial reality of dynamic spiritual forces, which are constrained neither by tripartite spatial nor temporal dimensions. To speak of higher beings working according to spiritual laws from "within" or from "without," the fourfold human being should not be conflated with physical laws by which, for instance, a bird shapes its physical nest from "within" on a tree branch, nor with the way a strong gust of wind can dislodge the nest from "without" or outside it.

7   We have long known that we grow and (to a large extent) heal primarily during sleep at night, but only recently have we been able to conduct empirical research also to document how we learn during the night by integrating (in reverse order) what we have experienced during the previous day, especially those experiences based in movement—both physiological motions and psychological e-motions. The implications for educational practices of this research cannot be overstated; they deserve separate discussion beyond the confines of this brief article.

8   D.H. Lawrence, *Fantasia of the Unconscious and Psychoanalysis and the Unconscious* (New York: Penguin Books, 1977), p.173.

9   Rudolf Steiner, *Karmic Relationships*, Volume VII, Lecture of 14 June 1924 in Breslau (London: Rudolf Steiner Press, 1973), p.117.

REFERENCES

D.H. Lawrence, *Fantasia of the Unconscious and Psychoanalysis and the Unconscious* (New York: Penguin Books, 1977).

Stefan Leber, ed., *Der Schlaf und seine Bedeutung: Geisteswissenschaftliche Dimensionen des Un- und Überbewussten* (Verlag Freies Geistesleben, 1996).

Michael Lipson, ed., *Sleep and Dreams: A Bridge to the Spirit* (SteinerBooks, 2003).

Richard Seddon and Jean Brown, eds., *The Wonders of Sleep: An Anthroposophical Study* (Wynstones Press, 2015).

Rudolf Steiner, *Course for Young Doctors*, GA 316 (Chestnut Ridge, NY: Mercury Press, 2008).

_____, *The Healing Process: Spirit, Nature, and Our Bodies*, GA 319 (Hudson, NY: Anthroposophic Press, 2000).

_____, *Karmic Relationships*, Volume II, GA 236 (London: Anthroposophical Publishing Company, 1956).

_____, *Karmic Relationships*, Volume VII, GA 239 (London: Rudolf Steiner Press, 1973).

_____, *Macrocosm and Microcosm*, GA 119 (Great Barrington, MA: SteinerBooks, 1968).

_____, *Man and the World of Stars*, GA 219 (New York: Anthroposophic Press, 1963).

_____, *Pastoral Medicine*, GA 318 (Hudson, NY: Anthroposophic Press, 1987).

_____, *Spirit as Sculptor of the Human Organism*, GA 218 (Great Barrington, MA: SteinerBooks, 2015).

_____, *The Occult Movement in the Nineteenth Century*, GA 254 (London: Rudolf Steiner Press, 1973).

_____, *The Sun Mystery and the Mystery of Death and Resurrection*, GA 211 (Great Barrington, MA: SteinerBooks, 2006).

Rudolf Treichler, "Sleeping and Waking as the Respiration of the 'I,'" in *Beiträge zur Einer Erweiterung der Heilkunst*, Heft I, Jan-Feb 1970, 23. Jahrg., pp.5–21 (translated by Douglas Gerwin and privately published).

Matthew Walker, *Why We Sleep: Unlocking the Power of Sleep and Dreams* (New York: Scribner, 2017).

Rest as Resistance:
A Social Aspect of Sleep

Linda Williams

Children's sleep differs from the sleep of an adult. Normally, adults process their waking experiences during sleep. Children cannot yet carry their waking experiences into sleep. Thus, in sleep they settle into the general cosmic order without taking their physical experience into the cosmic order. Through proper education, we must bring children to the point that they can carry their experience in the physical plane into what the soul-spirit does during sleep.[1]

One of my earliest and most favorite memories is of naptime. As a young toddler, in my urban Detroit home, naptime was part of the rhythm of a day that began with breakfast, followed by plenty of outdoor play in the backyard and in my grandfather's garden and garage workshop. As the sun reached its highest point, we were called in for lunch by our mother and, after lunch, ushered upstairs to our bedroom for naptime. My memory is of a hushed quiet (even though I shared a room with two other sisters), enfolded perhaps by a low hum from my mother. Under a favorite blanket and holding my doll, I remember feeling loved and secure, and especially acknowledged by the sunlight that streamed through our curtains. I felt the movement of sun and shadow as they passed over me and filled me with what I can only describe now as pure joy. Guided by these friends, my passage into sleep was smooth and unencumbered. My memory of this transition and how I was held echoes in my thoughts and in my heart as a teacher. The release of a young child into sleep is truly a holy moment.

This delicious memory of sleep contrasts sharply with my sleep memories as a school-age child and then as a young adult entering the larger circles of social life of school and work. The aspirational goals of my working class African American family were firmly implanted in all of us and the cultivation of sleep and rest quickly gave way to busy-ness, the business of life. Both of my parents worked full-time jobs out of the house and ran part-time entrepreneurial gigs in the evenings and on weekends. I remember falling asleep to the rhythm of my mother's typewriter and adding machine in the next bedroom as she completed accounting tasks for our neighbor's business. My father ran a television repair business out of our home, and we all learned to answer the phone as young office workers, taking and relaying messages during our free time. Even my elderly grandmother who lived with us still had commitments to the church and charitable societies to which she belonged, and meetings often required hours of preparation.

For me, the possible restful time after school became crowded with homework and piano lessons. Saturdays included private violin lessons and Girl Scout meetings. By high school and college, my siblings and I all had experience with all-nighters to produce exemplary projects for church or school or to study for tests. Having full-time and part-time jobs defined our existence from our teenage years onward. Sleep and rest became rest-stops—it seemed we all could be much more *productive* if we spent less time sleeping.

But, freedom to sleep, to rest in the rhythms of nature, is a human necessity, even a human right. Like access to clean air, pure water, and nutritious food, the ability to sleep deeply and securely is necessary for health and development—on the physical, soul, and spiritual level—for both children and adults. Thus, the need for rest, dreaming, and sleep has become one of the refrains in the chorus of social justice. Sleep and rest, therefore, is an equity issue. Who has the privilege of sleep and rest? Is the possibility for sleep, for rest, for dreams distributed equitably amongst all of us?

Most notably, Tricia Hersey,[2] artist, poet, theologian, and community organizer, recognized that the social forces that limit or deny rest must be resisted. Founder of the Nap Ministry, Hersey asserts that our entire (American) culture is "sleep-deprived and exhausted." What Rudolf Steiner identified as the forces of materialism, Hersey names white supremacy and toxic capitalism as the contributors to "grind" culture—a culture of over-doing, over-producing, and over-committing, attaching one's worth to productivity and consumption.

Hersey recognizes that sleep-deprivation is both a public health issue and a spiritual issue. She calls on all communities to help create spaces for rest, for daydreaming, for sleep. Her Nap Ministry helps me to wonder about how we can make our Waldorf schools more healthy for rest, daydreaming, and sleep—for both the children and the adults in our care. Questions we might consider include: How can we protect periods of rest for teachers and administrators? How do we structure our days and our buildings so that there are moments for quiet reflection and/or daydreaming or even meditation? How can we ensure that all of the adults and children in our community get the requisite hours of sleep so that they can be refreshed by spiritual forces?

Steiner notes, "Above all, we must be conscious of the primary pedagogical task, namely that we must first make something of ourselves so that a living inner spiritual relationship exists between the teacher and the children."[3] Making something of ourselves begins with the community of spiritual beings we engage with when we sleep. Resisting materialism by resting thoroughly could be our most helpful way forward.

ENDNOTES
1. Rudolf Steiner, *The Foundations of Human Experience* (Hudson, NY: Anthroposophic Press, 1996), p.42.
2. Tricia Hersey, *Rest Is Resistance: A Manifesto* (New York: Little, Brown Spark, 2022).
3. Op. cit., Steiner, p.44.

Healing Forces of the Night

Holly Koteen-Soulé

As modern human beings, the wakefulness required of us in daily life with our many roles and responsibilities can often make us feel fractured and fragmented at the end of the day. A good night's sleep can restore us, make us feel whole again, and heal a sense of fragmentation. This restoration of forces happens mostly without our conscious awareness. Sleep is a mysterious blessing we mostly take for granted unless it is disturbed or disrupted. How can the healing power of our nightly journey be enhanced if we understand the remarkable reciprocal alchemy between our waking life experiences and what transpires during sleep?

As an early childhood teacher and teacher educator, I often revisit the opening lecture of the training course that Rudolf Steiner gave to the teachers of the first Waldorf School. In that lecture he described the task of the Waldorf teacher as helping students to learn to "breathe" and "sleep." In my recent reading, I was struck by Steiner's focus on the opposite and complementary directionality of these two common, everyday human activities.

"We must be aware that when we teach children about this or that subject, we are actually working toward bringing the spirit-soul more into the temporal body and, at the same time in another direction, to bring temporality more into the spirit-soul."[1] In supporting a child's breathing, we are inviting the flow of substance from spirit realms into physical realms, and in supporting a child's sleep, we are encouraging the lifting up of earthly substance into the spiritual world.

For Steiner, breathing encompasses much more than the physical process of inhalation and exhalation. Human beings, Steiner explains, have two ways of relating to their surroundings: through conscious perception (via the senses and thinking) and through unconscious taking in of substances in highly dispersed states, as in breathing.[2] Children have not yet learned how to breathe in such a way as to fully connect their breathing with their nerve-sense system. When we help bring the child's breathing into relation with the nerve-sense process, we support the drawing down of the child's soul and spirit into physical life.

Children are also not yet able to reflect on and carry into sleep what they see, hear, and do during the day in the same way as adults process their daytime experiences. According to Steiner, what human beings acquire from the spiritual world comes to them during sleep. While we cannot give children spiritual content, we can help them gradually be able to carry their experiences from the physical plane into what their soul-spirit experiences in sleep.

When there is a rhythmic flow between physical/etheric and soul/spirit aspects of the human being, there is a greater harmonization of our earthly and spiritual natures. When these aspects are not in harmony, whether we are a child or an adult, our essential human capacities can be critically affected. That Rudolf Steiner asked the first Waldorf teachers to pay attention to the deeper significance of breathing and sleeping continues to be an unmistakable call for us to penetrate the deep mystery of these everyday activities in our own lives and those of our students.

The "breathless" pace of modern life and the current rise in sleep challenges for both adults and children underscore the need to deepen our understanding of these essential activities. These challenges bring up many related questions. In what way might sleeping challenges be linked to the lack of healthy breathing during the day? Both breathing and sleeping are an alternation of "taking hold" and "letting go." It is possible that, unless we can experience in a balanced and harmoniously alternating "taking hold" and "letting go" in the rhythm of our day, we may have trouble "letting go" into sleep.

Other related questions include: What can we learn from current trauma research about the role of rhythm in education and healing? In what specific ways can Waldorf teachers mediate the current cultural factors that seem to be affecting children's breathing and sleeping?

We can begin by recognizing that sleep is healing, not only for the body, but also for the soul and spirit. Understanding the deeper significance of breathing and sleeping can allow us to expand our understanding of healing to include the spiritual forces available for us to "draw down" during the day and those that help us process the daily experiences that we "offer up" at night in order to gain clarity and strength for our tasks in life.

Some Practical Suggestions

What we do during the day makes a difference to what can happen at night, and vice versa. The more we understand and consciously work with our journey through the night, the more we realize how inextricably these two polar aspects of our lives are entwined. Here are some suggestions as to how Waldorf teachers can prepare for the transition from day to night consciousness and more consciously embrace the forces that come from the night, allowing them to flow into the day that follows.

- *Filling Our Basket During the Day:*

Any kind of artistic activity helps prepare our imaginative faculties for the nighttime journey. Open-hearted listening to a child, a colleague, or a parent clears a space in the soul, as does tempering our own strong sympathies and antipathies or holding back quick judgments. Being aware of and acknowledging those moments when we encounter goodness, beauty, and truth during our day also belong in our basket.

Debriefing with our colleagues at the end of the school day and creating traditions for mealtime conversations with family members are additional means of distilling the precious essences of the day. Taking note of the unresolved questions that can benefit from being worked on during the night is important, especially if a faculty group is carrying a question together.

- *Preparing for Sleep:*

Going to sleep represents a threshold between two different states of consciousness. Releasing oneself from day consciousness is often not easy. It is supported by bodily rhythms and familiar rituals. Adults as well as children benefit from these rituals. The mood in which we do them, however, is critical. Reverence when we are tired may be more difficult to invoke, but it helps both adults and children release themselves from the rush of the day.

One of the things we learn from Steiner's various lectures on sleep is that we leave the power of thinking on this side of the threshold and carry only feeling and will into the night world.[3] So, the mood we take with us as we make the transition matters more than any thoughts we might be entertaining before going to sleep. Our review of the day should ideally proceed in pictures rather than words or admonitions. Gratitude for specific people and experiences also eases the release into sleep. Poetry, fairy tales, verses, or prayers offer picture language that will serve, like deep waters, to float our night boat.

During sleep, according to Steiner, we are engaged in a backward self-review of our day in which everything is evaluated in terms of our fundamental humanity.[4] Our effort, however meager, to do a backward review before sleep is a step toward greater effectiveness of this process.

Henning Köhler, in his book *Working with Anxious, Nervous, and Depressed Children*, uses the image of the Watcher on the Bridge to help us prepare our questions for our night-time helpers.

> Imagine yourself stepping onto a bridge as you fall asleep, and having had an opportunity to relate to your child's angel at the bridge's far end. Then picture a watchman posted there whom you have to justify your crossing to. What do you suppose he will ask you? His first question would be, "Are you bringing a clearly thought-out problem that concerns you deeply for the child's sake rather than a problem of your own?" His second question, one that may surprise you, would be, "Have you formed a really clear image of the child?" What does a "really clear image" mean? Under what conditions does that clear image form itself as one falls asleep? It happens gently as the result of having taken the trouble to observe the child keenly and lovingly at least once a day and to do so, as Rudolf Steiner put it, "with reverence for the child."[5]

- *The Moment of Waking:*

During the day our experience of the spiritual world is muted. This allows us to consciously develop our individual capacities. At night our experience is cosmic and manifold. This change of perspective allows us to take difficult questions into sleep and wake up with fresh forces and new inspirations. Besides reviewing the past day during our sojourn in the spiritual realms, we also encounter what is coming toward us from the future. Although we may not remember what we experienced, pausing intentionally as we emerge from the spiritual world in the morning may allow something unexpected and surprising to be grasped. Moral impulses come from the spiritual world during sleep. In a certain sense, every time we put a question at night to the spiritual world concerning our moral development, we receive guidance in response.

- *Letting the Night Forces Flow into the Day:*

Trust is the mood that allows us to release ourselves into the arms of the night and also enhances what we receive in our souls upon waking as potential healing for ourselves, for our students, and for our companions. What we glean from the night can over time re-enliven and reshape the way we think and live, sometimes subtly and sometimes with a strong sense of intuitive knowing.

Healing and Community

The longing that we hear in the world for greater wholeness could also be a call for greater integration of our day- and nighttime journeys. Perhaps we can more consciously recognize the way in which our nighttime spiritual community helps us sift through and extract the gold from our daytime adventures. Perhaps we can work more consciously with those whispered nighttime messages and allow them to help us and our earthly companions transform the dross of our day (or turn our straw into gold, as depicted in the Grimms' fairytale "Rumpelstiltskin"). Healing may be more of a communal and community activity than we realize!

In this age, according to Rudolf Steiner, when humanity's guiding spirits have stepped back to give us space for free action, our efforts to understand and work with the night forces can serve not only the needs and development of humanity, but also those spiritual beings closest to us.

> The stars once spoke to us.
> It is world-destiny
> That they are silent now.
> To be aware of the silence
> Can become pain for our earthly selves.
>
> But in the deepening silence
> There grows and ripens
> What we speak to the Stars.
> To be aware of the speaking
> Can become strength for the Spirit-Human.[6]
>
> *– Rudolf Steiner*

ENDNOTES

1. Rudolf Steiner, *The Foundations of Human Experience*, GA 293 (Hudson, NY: Anthroposophic Press, 1996), p.42.
2. _____, *The Mystery of the Trinity: Mission of the Spirit*, Lecture 4, "The Other Side of Human Existence," GA 214 (Hudson, NY: Anthroposophic Press, 1991).
3. _____, *Old and New Methods of Initiation*, Lecture 4, GA 210 (London: Rudolf Steiner Press, 1991).
4. _____, *Cosmosophy*, Vol. 2, Lecture 10, GA 208 (Clagiraba, Australia: Completion Press, 1997).
5. Henning Köhler, *Working with Anxious, Nervous, and Depressed Children* (Fair Oaks, CA: AWSNA Publications, 2001), p.7.
6. Rudolf Steiner, *Verses and Meditations* (London: Rudolf Steiner Press, 2004), p.97.

Sleeping to Awaken:
Sleep and Social Change

Vernon Dewey

Fundamentally, the Waldorf School does not want to educate, but to awaken. We aim to teach right breathing and the right rhythm between sleeping and waking.

— Rudolf Steiner

In the wake of World War I, the Waldorf school emerged as a force for social change. Today, when our own society hears calls for social change, including racial justice, pushing beyond gender binaries, and decolonization, it begs us to ask how Waldorf schools are faring amidst this social change? How do we engage? How do we engage with each other?

At its inception, the first Waldorf School did not pursue social change in a conventional manner. Instead, Rudolf Steiner emphasized that education had to do with teaching children to do two things properly: to breathe and to sleep. If this education was meant to be a force for social change, what might sleep (taking just one of these two activities) have to do with social change?

There is a certain relationship we have between our awareness of social issues and how "awake" we are. In fact, we even have a relatively newer word, "woke," which emerged from the African American community in the 1930s but has gained more widespread use in the last decade. The word itself has changed its meaning and changes with context, and its reception (whether heard positively or negatively) varies even more widely.

In many of his lectures, Steiner urges us all to awaken, but what he means by awakening is worth exploring.

Waldorf education is not a pedagogical system but an Art—the Art of awakening what is actually there within the human being. Fundamentally, the Waldorf school does not want to educate, but to awaken. For an awakening is needed today. First of all, the teachers must be awakened, and then the teachers must awaken the children and the young people.

An awakening is needed, now that mankind has been cut off from the stream of world-evolution in general. In this moment humanity fell asleep—you will not be surprised that I use this expression. They fell asleep, just as a hand goes to sleep when it is cut off from the circulation of the body.... Certainly, in the sphere of the intellect, tremendous progress has been made since the fifteenth century. But this intellect has something dreadfully deceptive about it.[1]

The kind of awakening that is usually called for in society is a form of intellectualism masquerading as wakefulness that Steiner characterizes as "intellectual dreaming." Intellectualism is not the task of Waldorf education. Our task is to awaken self-consciousness—spiritual consciousness. "The real question is: How is man to awaken the deepest nature within him, how can he awaken himself?.... How can we find the unearthly, the super-sensible, the spiritual, within our own beings?"[2] Our answer may come in a way similar to how the Hawaiian god Kukaohia'laka (commonly referred to simply as "Laka") received help in building a canoe.[3]

Laka came upon a tree of such strength and straightness that he deemed it excellent for a canoe. He prayed, felled the tree, but upon returning home, realized that he did not have the skill to shape the canoe. The next day he returned to continue working on the canoe but, to his surprise, saw the log was gone! Instead, he found the very same tree that he thought he had felled, standing back up where he had first found it. He felled the tree again, slept again, and again the next day found it upright and rooted. When this repeated itself a third time, he decided to seek advice from his grandmother.

The next day he returned to the tree, dug a ditch next to where the tree would fall, felled the tree, and hid in the ditch under the branches of the fallen tree. At night he overheard *menehune* (elemental spirit beings, akin to elves) talking together about lifting the tree. Laka caught two of the *menehune* and threatened their lives until the *menehune* made him a deal: The menehune would carve the canoe and haul it to the ocean for him if he prepared a shed for the canoe and offered them a feast. The next day Laka built a canoe shed next to the beach and laid out a feast of poi and shrimp. True to the word of the *menehune*, the next day Laka found a beautifully shaped canoe resting in its shed.

What might this story have to offer us?

1. *Having a vision*

The tree seems almost to be asking to be made into a canoe. What, in our own school circumstance, is asking to be done? Is there a ripe opportunity? There is a global cry for justice, for decolonizing, for diversity, but how do these ideas best manifest in each school? How do we recognize each school's unique calling?

2. Answering the call
Laka fells the tree. Here we have the first of Steiner's four essential qualities of the teacher: initiative.[4]

3. Humility
Laka realizes his own inadequacy at carving the canoe. It is interesting that it is only after felling the tree that Laka verbalizes his lack of skill as a carver.

4. Obstacle
The work of felling the tree is undone! Again! And again! It is at this point that Laka is repeatedly humbled. How many times have we set out to change something, to bring something to bear, only to have it seemingly be undone or never really come to fruition? It is worth reflecting on why that might be. It could be that the vision was of a personal nature, not what truly served the Being of the School. At other times, we may have the right initial vision, but that does not mean we alone are capable of fully shaping it.

5. Seeking wise counsel
Laka's first attempt to broaden his perspective is by reaching out to his grandmother, an elder. From the story it is unclear whether his grandmother gives him the plan or the plan arrives through their conversation. There seems to be wisdom in the way the story is told, leaving that part unknown, for what arises when any two people meet is quite mysterious. In our school life there is always value in seeking the counsel of a colleague and beholding what might then arise. When we are alone with a thought or an inspiration, it can have a tendency to move into

the clever, to live within the head, the intellect. When we open it into dialogue, then it travels further down into the rhythmic system where heart forces warm it and the lungs breathe it back and forth.

6. *Preparing for the night*

Equipped with inspiration born of dialogue, Laka prepares for the night. Talking story with his grandmother helps him prepare for what occurs at night, helps him witness the spiritual workings of night. He digs his ditch and waits, unknowing what will unfold. In this same way, we can work with our meditative life to settle into our question and wait, patiently, in a spirit of gentle beholding. The chalice has been formed and now we wait for spiritual beings to bestow their blessings.

7. *Catching the spirit*

Laka seizes two menehune and transforms their obstructing force into creative force. It may happen that we wake up in the middle of the night with a "Eureka!" moment, seizing upon a sudden inspiration. But more often than not our answers come quietly. They may arise in our meditation the next morning as images, a word, a phrase, a movement, or an impulse. We may not even notice it until later in the day when we are in the middle of a conversation or while completing some unrelated task. Regardless of when it comes, we make space within ourselves to be receptive, to listen, and to notice.

8. *Preparing the way*

The work is now underway, but we as a community must be prepared. Just as Laka needs to build a shed for his new canoe, we need to create a receiving space within the community for change. The purpose of building the shed is twofold: one, to help embody and integrate the change so that it does not sit like a piece of driftwood on the beach; two, to protect and honor this new gift. We create this space through conversation, through collaboration, so that all hands in the community help welcome it in. When we have done that, then all are invested in its success, all become guardians, stewards of the work. In our conversations with People of Color in our movement, often we have heard of the feeling of working in isolation, of the vulnerability of being a Person of Color, of the added scrutiny people from marginalized backgrounds feel in their classrooms, in their work. Cultivating a sense of belonging can begin in our meditative life, preparing for the night. We can take a colleague into our consciousness, with warmth of heart, "spirit beholding, heart-warm touching."[5] This act of taking interest will awaken in a stronger, deeper place the next day, nourished by spiritual powers.

9. *Gratitude*
Laka prepares a feast for the *menehune*.

Finally, it is important that we cultivate a continual spirit of gratitude. The spiritual world is ever active in our daily lives, but so seldom do we see and acknowledge its workings. On a daily level, we can practice giving thanks in the evening. Was there an insight we had that was particularly helpful? An interaction that shed new light onto something? An act of kindness that we received? An awakening to a blind spot that we didn't see before? When we take the time to give proper thanks for these moments, we help to nourish the spiritual powers that in turn feed us. On a larger scale, how do we give thanks when something is accomplished? When a teacher bravely and skillfully brings something new into the classroom? When the administration ushers in a new practice that cultivates more belonging and inclusion in our school? These too are the workings of spiritual beings and human beings who deserve thanks and praise.

To breathe and to sleep: These are two of our powers for social change. Expanding ourselves to each other and to the spiritual world, we awaken to the guiding activity of the spirit. We awaken to find our canoe, resting on the shore, with room for us all, ready to take us from where we are to where we wish to go.

ENDNOTES

1. Rudolf Steiner, *The Younger Generation*, Lecture II, GA 217 (Spring Valley, NY: Anthroposophic Press, 1967), p.23.
2. Ibid., p.28.
3. See Mary Kawena Pukui' and Caroline Curtis, *Tales of the Menehune* (Honolulu: Kamehameha Schools Press, 1985).
4. Rudolf Steiner, *Discussions with Teachers*, GA 295 (London: Rudolf Steiner Press, 1967), p.164.
5. _____, "Second Teachers Meditation" in *Toward the Deepening of Waldorf Education* (Hudson, NY: Waldorf Publications, 2017), p.109.

Sleep and the Chronology of Transformation

Vernon Dewey

I felt inspired to write the following after Nkem Ndefo, an organizational strategist who specializes in resilience and healing, mentioned the concept of "urgentocracy" in her keynote speech at the 2024 AWSNA Teachers Conference. How do we avoid imposing an urgentocracy on our schools without calcifying them due to a lack of change?

"What do we want?!"
"[*Fill in the blank*]!"
"When do we want it?!"
"NOW!"

If you have ever been to a protest, march, or rally, the above should be as familiar to you as homemade signs, megaphones, more pamphlets than you'll ever read, and that guy wearing suspenders covered in way too many buttons.

At first blush, the demand for change to happen now seems self-justifying. If something is wrong or unjust, should it not end immediately? Should not the new, better, more just thing begin as soon as possible?

Certainly, for some things immediate change is appropriate, but for most things the pace of change requires a different and more patient timeline. In our own institutions such as Waldorf schools, we have to remember that schools are composed of human beings. And for us as Waldorf educators who work daily with rhythms of human development, we know how important timing is when bringing experiences and concepts, and how the human being cannot grow, change, or transform according to a timeline other than its own. Our organizations are no different.

There is also such a thing as moving *too* slowly. One could easily argue that the racial reckoning following George Floyd's murder in 2020 is due in no small part to the glacial pace of positive change regarding racial equality and justice. "What happens to a dream deferred?" asks Langston Hughes in his famous poem, "Harlem."

> What happens to a dream deferred?
>
> Does it dry up
> like a raisin in the sun?
> Or fester like a sore—
> And then run?
> Does it stink like rotten meat?
> Or crust and sugar over—
> like a syrupy sweet?
>
> Maybe it just sags
> like a heavy load.
>
> *Or does it explode?*

For many in our movement, particularly (but not exclusively) for People of Color, as well as people of marginalized identities and young people, the pace of change in Waldorf schools regarding social issues has been too slow, a dream deferred. At the same time, for many in our movement, particularly (but not exclusively) those with more privileged identities and those who are older, the pace of change in Waldorf schools regarding social issues in recent years has been too fast, or at least hastily considered and implemented. All of this is normal, to be expected as it relates to the differences in unique personal clocks within our schools. And this is why we need to step beyond the individual with its own narrow rhythms and look to what we are trying to grow and transform in the school, the Being of the School.

In his collection of essays *Thy Will Be Done: The Task of the College of Teachers in Waldorf Schools*, Roberto Trostli quotes Rudolf Steiner's assertion that "wherever a group of people come together in the service of an ideal, a spiritual being is drawn to them." A Waldorf school is one clear example of this gathering of people around a shared ideal. How, then, do we come into contact with the Being of the School? Trostli answers:

> We can experience something about this being when we share our school's vision and values, participate in its customs and traditions, experience and understand our community better through the common ground of the school's biography.
> By working to perceive the character of the school, by finding the common language that unites the school, by seeking ways to recognize and utilize each other's gifts for the common good, the members of the College[1] can get to know the being of their school and invite it to participate in their work.[2]

When we are in this activity of spirit beholding, we can then become sensitive to the rhythm of unfolding that is being requested. Which sequence of events or images emerges and by which timeline? Are these in the short-term? Long-term? On what scale are these activities? Large? Small? Are they focused internally or externally? How does each image *feel*? To ask these questions and receive answers with our hearts is to use the soul-member most attuned to time. Our heads possess the power of picturing, imagining, but in regard to time everything is instantaneous. Thus, if you ask the head, the intellect, when something should be done, it is likely that the answer is "Now!" The heart lives in rhythm and is sensitive to the chronomic needs of the body. In a group, our collective heart may become sensitive to the chronomic needs of the collective, to the Being of the School. Essential to the sensing process of the heart is to give pause. We must pause and quietly attune ourselves to the collective feeling life, to the feeling life of the Being of the School.

Sleep is an activity that helps us put a pause on our waking consciousness, to loosen our narrow self-consciousness and dwell for a time amidst the collective, the Cosmic All. If we treat our daily sleep life with reverence, honoring its wisdom, then we better equip ourselves to enact "mini-sleeps" throughout the day. To listen, it has been said, is to fall asleep in the other. When we awaken to someone's needs, it is because we loosen ourselves from our ego and fall asleep into the other person's needs. We soften ourselves, loosen ourselves, enough to receive what they are sharing.

Here we can see that honoring our sleep life also means honoring our awakening life, the period of time just after sleep when we wake up.[3] Devoting attention to this period of time as individuals and as collectives can help us to awaken to ourselves, to each other, and to the Being of the School. Our questions can then become transformed from a scripted call and response to a living Parzivalian question:

"What ails thee [Being of the School]?"
"How may I [and members of the school] be of service?"

ENDNOTES

1 Although Trostli is speaking of the College of Teachers, the process described does not need to be confined to this particular grouping of individuals within a school.
2 Roberto Trostli, *Thy Will Be Done: The Task of the College of Teachers in Waldorf Schools* (Chatham, NY: Waldorf Publications, 2017), p.68.
3 Florian Osswald's essay on "Sleep and Rhythms," included in this collection, offers some helpful observations in this regard.

Sleep and Movement

Laura Radefeld

If all went well for us in childhood, we would have had many years of learning to move in every way possible, full of vigor, joy, and meaning: purposeful working activities, imaginative play, artistic expressive movement, articulate and skillful movement as a musician or skilled athlete, doing eurythmy. Meaningful movements all provide a path to inner balance and are equally important for children and adults.

Movement is essential for developing physical and inner balance, flexibility, fluidity, wakefulness, attentiveness, strength, and creativity. Distilled inner movement becomes the ability to be reflective, resourceful, and creative in our thinking. Inner movement also requires the achievement of inner quiet, the capacity to set all things aside and hold a space of inner solitude, balance, and peace.

Imagine the outer movement of childhood being transformed into capacities of inner movement and inner quiet. In our own development, an essential task is to develop the capacity to quiet ourselves, our urges, drives, thoughts, and movement in order to hold an inner space for listening and reflective, contemplative life. This can be challenging at any stage of life!

A key aspect of healthy bodily movement at every stage of life is to master the capacity of letting go—which can mean many things. In this context I will focus on letting go of our physical instrument and allowing ourselves to rest and/or sleep. This can be a complex process in our complex world. Letting go of the day, of our daytime preoccupations, in order to allow ourselves to meet the reality of the night is something we cultivate as a capacity throughout our life.

The process of letting go is one of releasing the day so that the forces available to us at night may help us. The evening hours can be seen as a time to prepare to relinquish the cares of the day to the forces of the night. Eurythmy can help with the process of letting go of the day.

A helpful exercise in this process is known as "A-H-Reverence." Gathering ourselves, we place our hands over our heart as if holding it in cupped hands. From here we slowly open our arms into the horizontal with an open "Ah" gesture, beholding the panorama of our day with love and appreciation or a feeling of reverence for all that has streamed toward us on this day. We lift this gesture of appreciation up above our head, arms outstretching in a large "Ah" gesture, and then draw back the shoulders with a pull toward the back space, opening the rib cage and feeling a wide "Ah" descending into the space behind, giving it over to the spiritual forces of the night.

Doing this sequence a few times opens a door into night consciousness and a sense of restfulness.

Resources
for further exploration into the nature and significance of sleep

compiled by Michael Holdrege

ANTHROPOSOPHICAL RESOURCES

The anthroposophically-oriented resources listed below cover many different aspects of sleep as it can be understood from a spiritual scientific perspective. They have proved very helpful to members of the Pedagogical Section Council in researching this topic.

Rudolf Steiner (2018). *The Night as a Wellspring of Strength: Sleep, Spiritual Encounters, and the Starry Firmament.* Spencertown, NY: SteinerBooks.

Rudolf Steiner (2003). *Sleep and Dreams: A Bridge to the Spirit.* Spencertown, NY: SteinerBooks.

Richard Seddon (2012). *The Wonders of Sleep: An Anthroposophical Study.* Stourbridge, UK: Wynstones Press.

Adam Blanning (2023). *Raising Sound Sleepers.* Edinburgh: Floris Books.

Audrey McAllen (1981). *Sleep: An Unobserved Element in Education.* Hudson, NY: Waldorf Publications.

Victor Bott (2004). *An Introduction to Anthroposophical Medicine.* Spencertown, NY: SteinerBooks, pp.46–57.

ADDITIONAL RESOURCES

The titles listed below have not been vetted by members of the Pedagogical Section Council but are representative of the wide-ranging literature now available on questions of sleep.

Michael Anch, et al. (1988). *Sleep: A Scientific Perspective.* Saddle River, NJ: Prentice Hall.

Stan Rodski (1923). *The Neuroscience of Excellent Sleep.* New York: Harper Collins.

Edzard Ernst (1999). *Sleep: Practical Ways to Restore Health Using Complementary Medicine.* New York: Sterling.

J. Paul Caldwell (2003). *Sleep: The Complete Guide to Sleep Disorders and a Better Night's Sleep.* Richmond Hill, Ontario, Canada: Firefly Books.

Matthew Walker (2017). *Why We Sleep: Unlocking the Power of Sleep and Dreams.* New York: Scribner.

Frances Jensen (2015). *The Teenage Brain.* New York: Harper Collins, pp.86–102.

Mission and Membership
of the Pedagogical Section Council (PSC)

The mission of the Pedagogical Section Council (PSC) of the School for Spiritual Science is to support the work of Waldorf teachers in our current times.

As a group of experienced Waldorf educators in North America belonging to the Pedagogical Section of the Anthroposophical Society, the PSC meets in person twice a year, as well as online between its in-person gatherings.

The work of the Council includes:

- Cultivating relationships with teachers, schools, and pedagogical and anthroposophical organizations
- Recognizing emerging phenomena in education
- Researching issues arising in the movement and in society at large and how these issues live in our places of work
- Communicating its findings through conferences, workshops, and publications
- Deepening the work through the Class Lessons

Currently active members of the PSC: Liz Beaven, Vernon Dewey, Douglas Gerwin, Michael Holdrege, Holly Koteen-Soulé, James Pewtherer, Laura Radefeld, Victoria Reyes-Cheng, Frances Vig, and Linda Williams.

Made in the USA
Middletown, DE
05 June 2025